Body Building

Building The Perfect Body With Simple Hints And Tips That Will Give You Dramatic Results

Introduction

I want to thank you and congratulate you for downloading the book, *"Bodybuilding: Building The Perfect Body With Simple Hints And Tips That Will Give You Dramatic Results"*.

This book has lots of amazing information on how to build the perfect body with simple hints and tips that will bring you dramatic results.

Have you ever thought of getting that "toned" look that everybody is after? And what crosses your mind whenever you come across the term "bodybuilding"?

Perhaps images of huge, heavy muscled bare-chested men and lean bodied ladies flexing their pectorals, massive biceps and triceps amidst tumultuous applauses from a fiery audience is what comes to your mind! That's pretty fine; only that it is part of bodybuilding; the professional one!

So what exactly is bodybuilding if the above is just part of it? Well, bodybuilding is the whole process you adapt to build your body from the ground up. And the good news is that adapting bodybuilding as your lifestyle will see you gain immense benefits ranging from fitness to personal health.

Therefore, understand what bodybuilding entails; know how to practice bodybuilding safely and obtain dramatic results, train consistently, have quality exercises, check on your diet and maintain a positive attitude and see amazing transformation in your physique.

This guide will help you demystify all your bodybuilding myths and give you some tips on adapting this exciting regimen.

Thanks again for downloading this book. I hope you enjoy it!

Table of Contents

Introduction

Table of Contents

The Basics of Bodybuilding

Bodybuilding: Why Bother?

Your Body Type: Its Place In Bodybuilding

Getting Started with Training

Exercises Targeting Individual Muscle Groups

Getting To The Next Level: Tips That Will Guarantee Massive Rapid Success

Conclusion

The Basics of Bodybuilding

Just as the introduction hinted, if you are to practice bodybuilding, it is critical that you understand what it is and what it entails. That's why tis first chapter is dedicated to just that.

What is Bodybuilding?

Bodybuilding refers to the process of growing and developing your body using exercises and diet. In other words, bodybuilding involves making use of proper progressive resistance exercises to regulate and develop your physique; exercises may vary from attaching weights to your bike to enhance acceleration, to increasing your gym time in order to strengthen your body muscles and improve your body shape. Furthermore, an athlete who is regularly bettering their agility and quickness for the field is also performing bodybuilding.
So what does it (bodybuilding) entail?
1: Bodybuilding uses gravitational force to oppose the force generated by your body muscles through eccentric or concentric contractions.
Let me explain:
An eccentric contraction occurs when your muscles encounter opposing greater force than they can generate; hence they elongate under such tension. Eccentric contractions are also called braking contractions and they take place when you perform such exercises as running downhill, descending on staircase or even during the downward motion of the pushups or squats.

On the other hand, concentric contractions refer to the shortening of your muscles as they generate opposing force. Most weight lifting exercises result to concentric muscle contractions; for instance, during the lifting phase of bicep curl or when running uphill.

2: Additionally, your diet also plays an important role in bodybuilding. Your diet must be constructed to help your muscles create mass and prompt muscle growth.

3: Another important aspect of bodybuilding is adequate rest; your muscles need time to heal and repair themselves. It is also during rest time that the muscle growth process is initiated.

In the long run, when you get into professional bodybuilding, employing 3 strategies of engaging in strength training, taking sufficient rest and specialized diet will help you build your body and increase your muscle size.

All in all, bodybuilding occurs when your muscles are severely stressed and forced to increase or elongate in order to adapt to the impeding force.

Note: Please note that bodybuilding is an art that is perfected through months of proper guidance, sincere efforts and utmost devotion. Nevertheless, when performed in the right way, bodybuilding will be of great benefit to you and make you feel rejuvenated at all times.

So why should you push yourself to engage in bodybuilding anyway? What's in it for you? Let me elaborate on that:

Bodybuilding: Why Bother?

You may practice bodybuilding for recreational purposes or simply as an avenue to increase your personal health and boost your self-confidence. Bodybuilding leads to a fit mind as well as a fit body. Once you make it your lifestyle, you may also take it a notch higher and do bodybuilding as a competitive sport, where you may gain international exposure and win many accolades. Some of the notable benefits of bodybuilding include the following:

1. **Improving Your Body Health**

✓ The risk of developing coronary heart disease is reduced through bodybuilding. When you exert more effort or consume energy, your heart gets exercised through the heartbeats. Through regular exercising, your heart muscles get strengthened.

Note: Sometimes the intensity of natural bodybuilding can have detrimental effects to your heart. For instance, lifting more than half your bodyweight may contribute to the risk of tearing your aorta. Therefore, it's prudent to undertake screening tests before doing any heavy lifting. Undertaking aerobic exercises such as biking or running also strengthens your heart and protects it against adverse effects of bodybuilding.
However, when considering taking part in long-term bodybuilding activities that may involve lifting heavy weights, always consult your doctor before beginning.

✓ Engaging in such physical activities as aerobic exercises and weight training gives you a good opportunity to reduce and control high cholesterol, obesity and high blood pressure.

✓ Bodybuilding also strengthens your bones. How does it do that? Well, weight-bearing activities and intense body movements have long-term effects of stimulating production of signals that increase your bone mineral density. When your bones are strained, your body responds by making your bones stronger. Normally, aging leads to a decrease in bone strength that may make them become brittle and easily prone to fracture. Bodybuilding increases your bone density to the point of lessening the risk of osteoporosis and arthritis. As you go on exercising in old age, you can easily reverse your bone loss tendencies.

✓ Bodybuilding can help increase your muscle mass. So how does it do that? Well, when you undertake long-term bodybuilding exercises, your body becomes stronger and leaner. Usually, as you age, you start losing muscle mass and strength. Bodybuilding leads to increased production of anabolic hormones. For instance, compound exercises like deadlift and squat enhance production of HGH (growth hormone) and testosterone that transforms your body by helping you maintain your muscle mass and strength, thereby keeping you bigger, stronger and more self-confident.

2. Increasing Your Strength And Flexibility

By training through the full range of motion, your joints become very flexible and can withstand any stress. Additionally, you are able to do away with chronic pains and aches such as back aches and any pains in the joints. Also, bodybuilding helps you to gain strength to lift heavy loads; since your level of endurance and balance are also enhanced.

3. Weight/Fat Loss

Bodybuilding entails lots of physical activity. When you think about it; this increases your body's energy demands, which essentially means that your body will have to source for the energy from somewhere. If you maintain your normal diet (assuming you don't overeat), you will essentially be creating a calorie/energy deficit when you exercise thus prompting your body to seek alternative sources of energy. The immediate source of this energy (now that the dietary calories are not enough) is stored body fat. This ends up burning and reducing your stored body fat reserves, which could end up making you to lose weight (if that's your goal). Moreover, the fact that bodybuilding results to improved muscle composition means you will essentially have a generally higher metabolic rate i.e. your body will burn more fat even while you are at rest.

4. Gaining A Better Posture And Better Looking Body

Regular training helps you to increase your muscle size, burn body fat and develop a better body. In fact, your musculature becomes very impressive. Furthermore, by regularly training your core and back muscles, you can prevent any cases of muscle imbalances and fix any disproportion. You are likely to end up with a straight back giving you a more attractive look.

5. Making You Happier

Since bodybuilding is a sport, it stimulates your body to secrete endorphins hormones, which reduces pains and makes you feel happier and better. This is best applied in stressful moments, when having mood swings or when suffering from depression. Bodybuilding exercises can prevent all these cases.

Now that you are aware of the perks that come with bodybuilding, I know you are excited to get started. So where should you start? Well, for starters, you need to understand that bodybuilding is highly personalized. Therefore, what may be ideal for one person may not be ideal for you. This doesn't mean you need something highly specialized though; you can start from somewhere i.e. knowing your body type. That's what we will be learning next.

Your Body Type: Its Place In Bodybuilding

Basically, not all bodies are created equally. There are three body types: the mesomorph, the ectomorph and the endomorph. You must know your body type in order to tailor your training program and set accurate but attainable goals to enable you succeed. Below are some features of these body types:

Ectomorph

This is a skinny guy. As an ectomorph, you are likely to have lean stringy muscles and small joints.

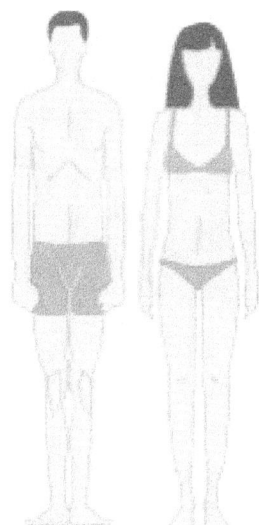

If you are an ectomorph's, you are likely to have these traits:

- Long limbs

- Thin build with small shoulders

- Slender hips and clavicles

- Flat chest

- Fast metabolism

Note: Gaining weight as an ectomorph is likely to be hard, due to having a fast metabolism, which consumes calories very quickly. Therefore, you must consume a higher amount of calories in order to gain weight. Your workout sessions must be intense but very short and ensure to always use supplements. Moreover, ensure you eat before sleeping to avoid muscle catabolism at night.

Mesomorph

This is a naturally athletic physique characterized by large muscles and bone structure.

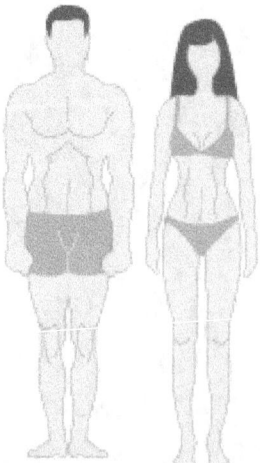

As a mesomorph, gaining and losing weight is very easy for you. Some of the traits of a mesomorph are:
- A hard, strong and rectangular shaped body

- Well-built muscles (long and round muscle bellies)

- Wide clavicles and a narrow waist

- Thinner joints

- Gains fat and muscle more easily than ectomorph

With mesomorph body, bodybuilding gains are easily seen, especially if you are a beginner. However, gaining fast is faster than ectomorphs and therefore your calorie intake must be watched. When training, always combine your weight training with cardio exercises.

Endomorph

This is a solid, soft and short body with thick limbs.

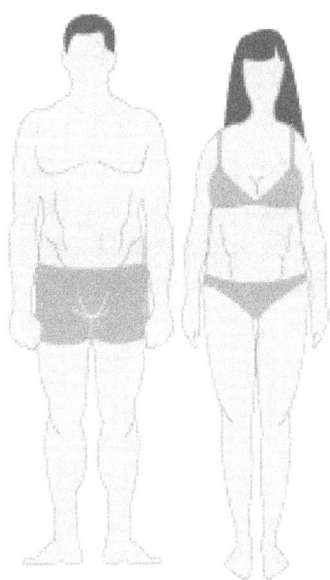

As an endomorph, your upper legs are strong. Endomorph traits are as follows:

- ✓ Thick rib cage and joints

- ✓ Wider hips than clavicles

- ✓ Short body and round physique

- ✓ Undefined muscles

Normally, endomorphs easily gain body fat because they have a slow rate of metabolism. Ensure to train with weights as well as cardio, but avoid supplements especially when you have a high intake of proteins. Due to your stronger upper leg muscles, leg exercises such as squat are best for you.

In addition to knowing your body type, it is important that you understand that genetics limit what you can easily achieve and what you are naturally gifted with. For instance, your muscle shape, bone structure and metabolism rate are determined by genetics and your training will require a lot of extra effort to realize any gains. Sometimes you may find your body type is a combination of the above. Just let your training and diet be guided by your body type in order to excel at bodybuilding.

However, remember bodybuilding is a self-discovery regimen and you must dedicate a good part of your time to it. The following section handles some of the beginners' exercises to get you oriented to bodybuilding. Therefore, it's time to work out your body. Let's dive into it straightaway!

Getting Started with Training

As you get started, keep the following in mind:

1: Bodybuilding works on the principle of injuring your muscles by lifting weights to build muscles. When perfectly done and on the appropriate scale, bodybuilding undertakes damage repair between workouts to enable your body to adjust and develop new muscles in order to muddle through future exercises.

2: Distinguishing between lifting for muscle and lifting for strength is very important in order to know how to carry out your exercises. This is because lifting big weights may certainly lead to increase in your muscle mass but you won't receive the results as fast as when you do it for bodybuilding specifically.

For instance, a rep range of 4-6 reps is ideal for increasing your strength. Your body learns to get stronger in anticipation of any lifts of this weight; that it may be subjected to in the future. On the other hand, for improving your muscle mass, a rep range of 8-12 reps is necessary to cause microscopic tears in your muscles. When repaired, these tears allow new muscles to be built.

3: Please note that for you to start achieving your dream body, your strength level must be worked to a certain level. You can hasten this process by increasing the weight in your last set of an exercise so that only 4-6 reps are done. Once your strength gets to better levels, work out for maximum muscle increase. For bigger weights, aim for 8-12 reps in your majority part of your sets and keep adding weight as you improve gradually.

4: Also always take advantage of the power of the negative rep. Try lowering the weight gradually and getting full control in order to push your muscles further to a higher level. Let your negative rep take at least twice as more time as the positive one, to have a dramatic increase in blood flow and lead to muscle increase.

5: Always warm up to prevent injuries and unlock your full potential. You may warm up using static or dynamic stretching exercises. In static stretching, hold the intended position (e.g. squat position) for 15-30 seconds. While with dynamic stretching, take controlled movements through various ranges of motion. You can do such exercises as light kicks, shoulder rolls or twists as forms of dynamic stretching. You can do a twist as follows:

Performing a Twist

- Get a weight plate.

- Sit on the ground and let your knees and hips bend at right angles.

- Keeping your back straight, hold the weight plate straight in front of you (ensure your torso is at 45° to the ground.)

- Twist your torso to the left, going as far as you can.

- Repeat the motion, but in the opposite direction.

- Then do 3 sets of 8-12 to master it.

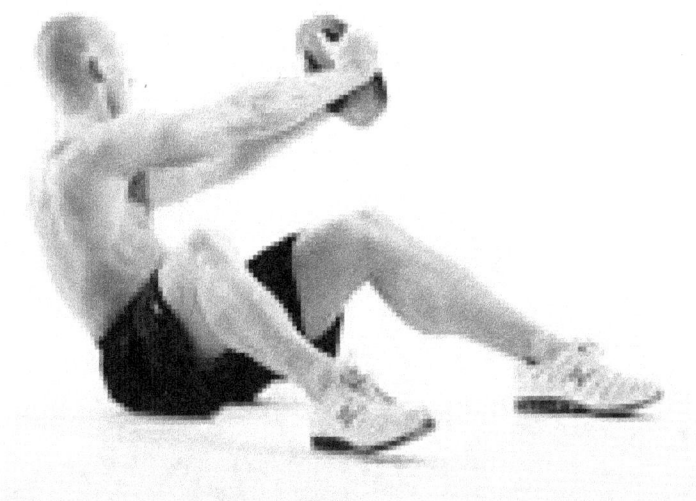

Before beginning on the exercises, it is important to observe some rules of etiquette, especially while at the gym. A few of these rules are as outlined below:

- Bring a towel each and every time, to wipe off the equipment and machines you make use of.

- Avoid resting for long periods of time on machines that others are waiting to use.

- Replace all the used dumbbells and barbells and rerack all the weight.

- Do not bring your cellphone into the training room to avoid unnecessary distractions.

When exercising, use free weights and not machines to get a full range of motion and build smaller controlling muscles to support your strength generally. You can use machines as supplements to help you in carrying out advanced techniques. The following are some of the exercises you can practice:

Squats

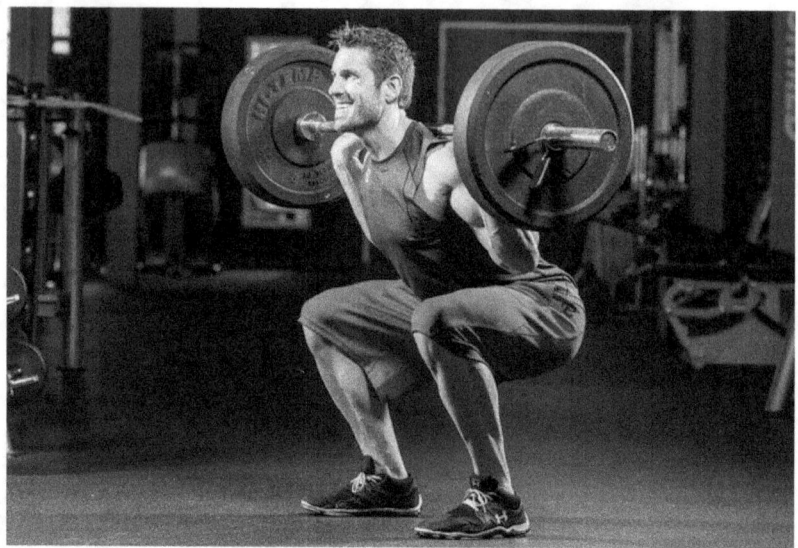

This is normally referred to as the king of all exercises because it targets many body parts with a greater focus on your lower back muscles, glutes and legs. That's not all; it engages more motor units and muscle mass, and is good for burning body fat.

Tip: When learning squats, avoid using lifting belt but start using bodyweight alone until you master the squatting technique.

Here is how to do squats:

- Put your feet about shoulder width apart and flat on the ground. Let your knees bend as you get near the bar whose height is already adjusted to your own height; ensure your weight is kept on your heels. Your weight should not be distributed to the ball of your or toes. If your feet are straight ahead, your knees are likely to cave in; therefore let your feet be inclined a little. Also, avoid standing with your feet further than shoulder width to prevent stressing the medial collateral ligament and knee cartilage. Your feet shouldn't be too close to avoid stressing your toes.

- Move your shoulders below the bar. The bar should be across your shoulders' back.

  Placing the bar over your trapezius muscles, grab it with your hands at a comfortable spot (about 15cm away from your shoulders); the bar should be weightless to enable you master the motion first. Lift and remove the barbell from the rack and move one step forward, so that the rack doesn't cause unnecessary motion interference.

- While looking straight ahead, with your heels on the floor, your chin up and your back straight, bend your knees and gradually lower your hips just like "siting" on a chair. Begin by going as far as you can to the chair seat level; with practice you'll be able to get there.

- Let your lower back remain in a neutral position and pull in your abs. If your back curves slightly, don't worry. Maintain your chest and head up to counter this as much as possible. For a full range motion, ensure your thighs are parallel to the ground.

  Unlock your body power by having tightened abs throughout the movement; your body helping you manage the weight, which should remain distributed in your feet and upper thighs.

- Maintain a proper and safe form, push up off your heels and lift the weight. Let all your body parts be actively involved as your legs are straightened and gradually but steadily move up. Your glutes should be exercised to give you power as you move up without letting your spine curve.

Note:

1: Your spine should remain upright only with your slight natural curve. Even if you get tired, do not bend your back at all. Never do a rep if it becomes impossible to do it without your back arching.

2: Always keep your knees in position. They should not pull while squatting. Bend the knees but they should remain almost in the same position by keeping them outward but not pushing through the toes. Also, your knees should not extend beyond your toes, to avoid causing muscle damages.

3: The bar should never rest on your neck base but on your upper shoulder muscles. Always have a wider grip of the bar.

- Breathe in as you drop down; while coming back up, breathe out to make use of your body's natural rhythm for smooth movement of the squat.

Bench Press

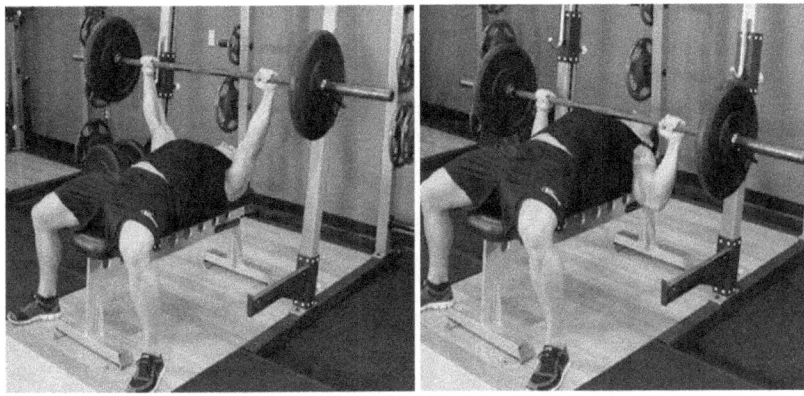

This exercise is aimed at developing your upper body strength; it targets your front shoulders, your chest, your back and your triceps. Follow the following steps to perform a bench press:

- Lie on your back on the flat bench and let your eyes be under the bar. With your feet flat on the ground, raise your chest and compress your scapula.

- With your little finger on your bar's ring marks, and using a full grip, keep your wrists straight and hold the bar in your palm's base.

- Take a big breath, straighten your arms and remove the bar from the rack. Keep your elbows locked and move the bar over your shoulders.

- While your forearms remain vertical, tuck your elbows at 75° and lower the bar to your mid-chest; as you hold your breath at the bottom.

- Then press the bar from your mid-chest to way over your shoulders as your butt remains on the bench. While at the top, lock your elbows and breathe.

Tip: Ensure you don't throw the weight at all; just maintain full control and go gradually.

- After bench pressing five reps, rack the weight by pressing the weight away from your chest up to when your elbows are locked. Let the bar move horizontally to your power rack from over your shoulders as you aim for power rack's vertical parts. Then bend your elbows lowering the bar in the uprights after hitting the vertical parts.

Note: Always tuck your elbows at 75° whenever you lower the bar; avoid flaring your elbows at right angles. Moreover, ensure the bar doesn't move vertically, for proper form bench pressing; let it move diagonally from your mid-chest across your shoulders.

Deadlifts

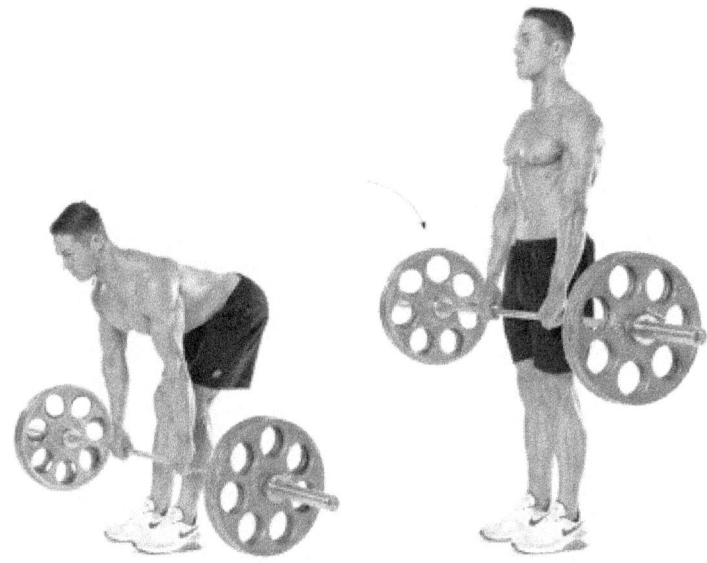

So what can deadlifts do for you?
Well, generally, deadlifts help in building the core strength
that supports other muscle groups within your body. This
exercise targets your squads, glutes, arms, abs and even your
back. It's also argued that practicing deadlift helps you get
mentally stronger. And since it strengthens your back and the
surrounding muscles, deadlift is also preferred for carrying
out preventive and rehabilitative works in your body.
Follow the steps below to do this exercise:

- Begin by putting the bar on the floor.

- Get closer to the bar; let your mid-foot stand under the
  bar, but don't let your shins touch. Keep your feet hip-
  width apart and let your toes protrude out.

- Narrow your legs to about shoulder-width apart; keep
  your arms vertical from the front view and let them
  hang outside your legs.

- Let your knees bend forward and proceed in the same motion until the bar is touched by your shins; keep the bar over your mid-foot and don't move it.

- While doing all this, keep your back straight but avoid dropping your hips and compressing your scapula. You shouldn't move the bar.

- Taking a big breath and then hold the bar; while keeping the bar against your legs, stand up without shrugging at the top. At this level, you have completed one deadlift with your knees and hips locked.

- Next, push your hips back and return the bar to the floor without bending your knees.

- After a second's rest, do the second rep; ensure the bar doesn't bounce off the floor. Ensure it is pulled from a still state.

- With sets of five reps every workout, you should be able to excel at this exercise.

Dips

This strength training exercise targets your deltoids, pecs,
rhomboid muscles and triceps. Your body must have a solid
base of strength for you to perform a dip. The idea is to lift
your whole body up and down. Therefore, you need two
parallel bars (dip bars). You train by lowering your body to
the point where your shoulders get below your elbows, and
subsequently pushing yourself upwards until your arms
straighten again.

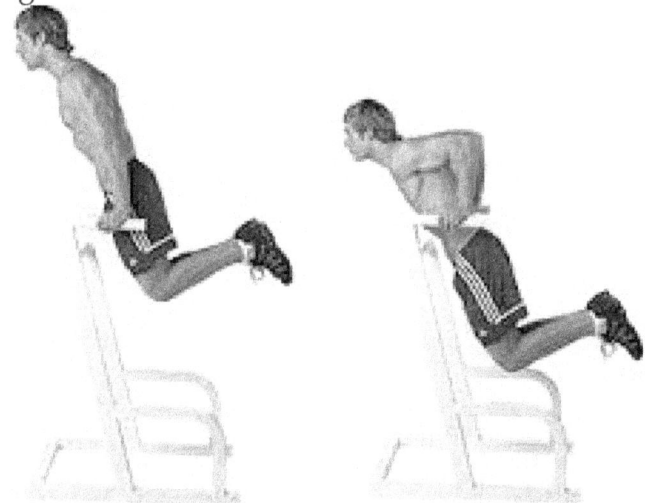

When performing a dip, your shoulders should not roll
forward or shrug at all; rather, they should be kept back and
down.
Note: Dips are not as effective as squats, for building strength
and muscle.
Perform dips using the following steps:

- Get two dip bars; they should be fixed, stable and
  parallel. Your gym may have a dip station; use it.

- Hold the bars, jump up and balance yourself by locking
  your elbows.

- Then bend your arms and lower yourself. Let you're your torso lean forward gently.

- Straighten your arms and lift yourself until you get to the starting position.

- Maintain balance by keeping your shoulders above your arms and having your elbows locked.

- Should you find it hard to do a single dip, start doing negatives. You may start by missing the way up and just do the way down only. While holding the dip bars, jump up, straighten your arms and lower yourself gradually to the point where your shoulders get beneath your elbows. Step on the floor and jump back to the starting position. After successfully completing 10 negatives, try a single dip.

With several repetitions, dips should work for you as fast as possible.
Note:
1: Always keep your abs and elbows tightened up and your body should be balanced while lifting and lowering yourself.
2: Instead of adding weight, just go very slowly. As you lower your body with your abs tightened, move ridiculously slowly to allow your body to recruit all muscles in your shoulders, chest and triceps.

The above are some of the compound exercises, which you can start with and have a complete full body workout in a shorter time. However, it is also good to add to your training program some of the exercises that focus on individual groups of muscles. Only do this if you have gained a lot of confidence with the compound exercises. The next chapter discusses one of these exercises.

Exercises Targeting Individual Muscle Groups

There are very many exercises targeting specific muscle groups; these exercises can be applied whenever you want to concentrate on an area that is troublesome. Also, sometimes other areas may be injured and you feel like trying a separate muscle group may not affect your efforts negatively and put your body at risk. Some of these exercises are:

- The bar raises - targets deltoids

- The incline curls - focuses on the biceps

- The cable pulldowns – concentrates on the triceps

- Fly's – hitting on the chest muscles etc.

This guide discusses fly's exercise.

The Dumbbell Chest Fly's

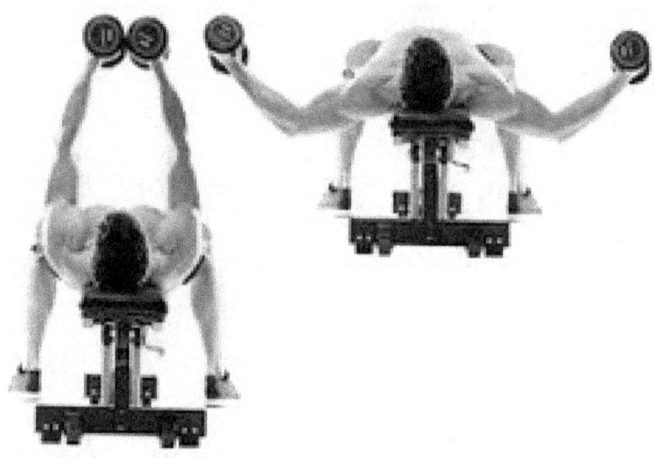

Dumbbells have an added advantage over fixed machines in performing fly's exercises especially because they incorporate more stabilization fibers and muscle mass.

This exercise targets the pectoral muscles, even though some of your biceps, forearm and shoulder muscles may be used. You can perform this exercise through the following steps:

- **Starting point:**

  - Select your dumbbells; this should be a weight load that you can easily do full motion with.

  - Get an elevated bench or flat surface that can take your full body length.

  - With dumbbells in your hands, lie on your back on the bench. Your back and head should be flat and your feet should be firmly stepping on the ground.

- o Let your arms straighten out, slightly bending at almost 5-10°.

- **Performing the upward phase:**

  - o Contract your pectorals. Act as if you are gripping an object in their midst; like a pencil.

  - o Raise your arms as if you want to cuddle a barrel without allowing your elbows to excessively bend.

  - o Your feet should not come off the ground while your lower back should not curve excessively.

When the dumbbells come into close contact over your head; that is a complete motion.

- **Performing the downward phase**

  - o Gradually lower your arms without having your elbows bend too much.

  - o Your dumbbells should not bounce back down.

  - o After finishing the reps, let your dumbbells come to your body's center and take them gradually to the end of motion.

- Raise your feet off the ground and put them on the bench while bending your knees to make this exercise target the pectoral muscles.

- When descending downwards, keep going until you feel a distinct stretch in your pectoral muscles. Wait for a little while and then go back up.

With all the above exercises, you can draft a workout schedule and begin your weight training journey. Set your weight training goals and dedicate your time and effort to it. Note: Remember that training for quality is always better than training for quantity. Therefore, hold short but intense training sessions; that are just enough to work your muscles as envisaged.

With the techniques we've discussed so far, I can bet that you've been seeing tremendous improvements in your body if you've been implementing them. To take this training to the next level, we will now discuss some tips to catapult your bodybuilding efforts to the next level.

Getting To The Next Level: Tips That Will Guarantee Massive Rapid Success

As seen earlier on, bodybuilding is a progressive regimen that you can start at any age. Likewise, as a beginner, your success in bodybuilding will be as a result of your careful attention to the following points:

- Capitalize on doing compound movements. Focus on the basic movements first and avoid trying any other possible exercise you see. Compound exercises normally target a muscle group simultaneously. Such movements constitute extending or flexing at least two joints. Some of the best exercises to try out are the shoulder press, squat, Lat pull downs and bench press.

  The bench press works your shoulders, triceps, chest and to a small degree, biceps. The hamstrings and the squads are worked by the squat exercises at the same time; while the shoulder press works on your triceps and shoulders.
  Using a maximum 2-3 per training day will be very helpful.
- Sticking to free weights will help you build a solid foundation of muscle mass. In particular, barbells and dumbbells will greatly help you build your muscle mass as a beginner.

- Always draft a training program and adhere to it. Formulating a strict routine and sticking to it will be of great benefit to you; your personal trainer or your mentor in bodybuilding can help you come up with a program. The program must clearly state the exact exercises you need to do, the associated number of sets and reps (a complete execution of a particular exercise) per set (a combination of any number of reps of a particular exercise). A program outlines the exact things you do whenever you go into a gym.

- It is important to train each muscle group every week; avoid very few workouts. However, do not overdo it by training every day.

- Make every attempt to learn the correct form of each exercise. Begin with lower weights and progress as you learn the right form of each exercise. Then start increasing the weights periodically. Take note of how much you lift on each exercise and gradually increase the weight fortnightly to increase your strength and result to muscle gain.

- As you begin using big weights, consider using safety belts for your lower back protection. This is because you are likely to develop back problems if you don't take extra caution.

- Your diet should consist of a lot of proteins, fruits and vegetables. You can get proteins in fish, chicken, eggs, nuts and dairy products. It is mostly recommended that you take 1 gram of protein per pound of your body weight to get the best results. You may add protein shake if you find it hard to consume enough proteins daily. Also, remember vitamins and minerals are needed by your body. As you do that, ensure to always avoid junk food and consume fast absorbing carbohydrates just after exercises; these are foods that are rich in sugar and flour. Finally, avoid being hungry; eat as often as possible, with 4-5 meals per day that are taken every 3-4 hours; and take plenty of water.

- Ensure that you eat more calories than you burn in order to build your muscles. You can calculate your Basal Metabolic rate (BMR) using this calorie calculator. Essentially, if you have an active lifestyle, you need more calories; but if your lifestyle is sedentary then you need fewer calories.

- Ensure to rest sufficiently to allow your body enough time to repair and build muscles. Normally, when sleeping, your body releases the HGH (growth hormone) during the REM part of sleep, which initiates muscle growth. Therefore, always avoid sleep deprivation as well; aim for 10 hours of sleep, and sleep for a minimum of 8 hours a night. However, do not exercise every single day; your routine should consist of 3-4 workouts per week. Spend the rest of the days resting and recovering. Also, spend 1-2 minutes to recover in between sets. If you take a longer resting time, you will be developing strength. However, the short recovery time allows you to maintain blood flow to your muscles; your strength drops set after set as more and more muscle stimulation is achieved. It is important to bear in mind that if you don't allow yourself recovery time, your muscles will experience improper healing and make you train exhaustively.

- Be consistent and patient. Muscle gains take a long time to be noticed. Therefore, don't miss too many workouts and train for the long haul.

- Keep challenging your body to get stronger as time goes; you must get stronger. Therefore, always stress your muscles by giving them extra loads and see the reaction.

- Exercise balancing your body part training. Your major muscle groups such as shoulders, back, squads and chest require 9-15 sets in a week while minor muscle groups such as calves, hamstrings, triceps, biceps and abs require 6-9 sets within a week.

While training, note that bodybuilding is not as complicated as it may appear. By observing the above basics and quality suggestions, you are able to get on track and progressively make great gains. However, another important point to note is that your body type matters a lot. This is because your body type determines how you physique evolves as you train.

Conclusion

Getting started with a bodybuilding regimen is always the trickiest thing. However, embrace bodybuilding and perfect it progressively as you reap immense benefits of body fitness and personal health. Just be consistent, patient and passionate about bodybuilding and train properly while adhering to your program.

Thank you again for downloading this book!
I hope this book was able to help you to understand the ins and outs of bodybuilding and how to use the information you've learnt to do something.
The next step is to implement what you have learnt.

Finally, if you enjoyed this book, would you be kind enough to leave a review for this book on Amazon?

Click here to leave a review for this book on Amazon!

Thank you and good luck!